Essential Oils 101
Oils and the body human

Written by Reiki Master Teacher, *Jane Howe*

Introduction:

A little history.

Essential oils and plant extracts have been woven into history since

the beginning of time and are considered by many to be the missing link in

modern medicine. They have been used medicinally to kill bacteria, fungi and

viruses and to combat insect, bug and snake bites in addition to treating all kinds of

mysterious modalities.

Oils and extracts stimulate tissue and nerve generation.

Essential oils also provide exquisite fragrances to balance mood, lift

spirits, dispel negative emotions and create a romantic atmosphere.

(Cite: 2011 Essential oils Desk reference 5th edition, Life Science Publishing)

Defining Essential Oils,

More specifically,what are essential Oils? They are natural components of shrubs, herbs, flowers, weeds and trees that possess medicinal properties.

How are they obtained? The plants, and alike   are put through a cold press process,   distilled and then bottled for use.

How are they used?

Inhalation or, Aromatherapy

Essential oils can be placed in misting diffusers, usually distilled water is placed in the diffuser reservoir and the essential oil droplets are added to the water. The diffuser creates a cool mist infused with the aroma of the essential oils . Atomizing the room air with the scent. As mentioned above each essential oil provides a different health benefit, so choosing the correct oil to support your desired outcome is important.

More on specific oils and the   system they support.

Topical Usage is applying essential oils directly on the skin. It is not limited to supporting a skin issue, but the absorption of the oil through the skin helps support overall health.

   One of the most rapid ways to get the oils into the body is placing the oil on the soles of the feet. The skin on the sole is much more thin then most of the skin of the body promoting ease and speed of absorption.

From the time of application the oils reach the bloodstream in less than 10 minutes.

Ingestion or Swallowing

Essential oils can be ingested or easier said eaten. Jasmine oil is the only essential oil that I know of to be poisonous when consumed. However Jasmine can be inhaled or used topically without ill effects. The length of time for essential oils to reach the bloodstream via ingestion is still being researched.

* ALWAYS READ LABELS TO ENSURE YOUR OWN SAFETY*

Often the chosen application of ingestion is placing the essential oils in a vegetable capsule and diluting the more hot oils (spicy like oregano, cinnamon, clove etc) with a carrier oil such as organic coconut oil or organic extra virgin olive oil.

Chapter 2

The Integumentary System

The integumentary system more commonly known as the skin.

Organ is the skin . The skin is the Largest organ of the entire body

Major components   of the integumentary system:

The epidermis is the outermost layer of the skin and the body's first line of defense against injury and pathogens.

It provides a waterproof layer and it also helps to control body temperature by opening and closing the pores and also using the hair follicles to trap heat.

When one experiences *goosebumps* this is what is happening.

  The Dermis is the second or middle layer of the skin. It houses the sweat glands, oil glands and hair follicles. It contains collagen and elastin which aids in keeping the skin flexible and strong. The dermis holds the majority of the body's water, provides blood to the epidermis and helps control body temperature as well.

The subcutaneous layer is the innermost layer. It is a pathway for nerves and blood vessels, from the dermis to the muscle tissue . It helps to regulate body temp as well, and protects the musculo-skeletal system from damage.

Sudoriferous sweat glands help by secreting water to the surface to aid in cooling the body down by the evaporation process of the water. Also another kind of sweat gland known as apocrine sweat glands, continuously secrete a fatty sweat associated with hair follicles into the tubule of the gland. Aiding the body also in ridding salts and impurities.

Sebaceous oil glands Help to keep skin lubricated and more supple to help prevent a break in the skin's integrity protecting you from an array of issues, including but not limited to pathogen entry into the body.

Pores are a gateway to the surface of the epidermis, they help control temperature buy opening and closing, IE. closing (goosebumps) when it's cold and opening up or dilating ,when it's hot to allow sweating etc. Pores also provide an exit for sweat, salts and impurities to the exterior.

Hair Follicles major purpose is to trap heat by standing straight up in response to cold, as detected when one experiences goosebumps.

Chapter 3

Some of the more commonly known skin issues

Dry chapped or chaffing of the skin. Remember that the skin is the first barrier and protection of the body so a break in the skin's integrity caused by one of the above can be quite a problem even if it seems like no big deal. It's allowing pathogens, bacteria , virus, etc. a free ticket to enter. This can open the door to a plethora of illness. So keeping the skin supple and soft , so it does not easily break or open is key in prevention.

Eczema ,though the exact cause of eczema is unknown , it is thought to be an immune response to an irritant , IE an allergic type response. There seems to be a trend in families that are prone to allergies and asthmatic illnesses and having eczema. Eczema is characterized by dry,rough very itchy skin patches. The skin cracks and bleeds, making one susceptible to skin infections, not to mention how agonizing it is to experience.

Psoriasis is similar to eczema in the sense that it too is an autoimmune response to an allergen/ irritant. It causes a rapid build up of skin cells which in turn results in flaking, scaling and inflammation of the skin.

Chapped and dry skin as a result of a plethora of causes but the most common are exposure to extreme climate from high heat and sun to frigid temperatures and wind chills. The outer layer of the epidermis skin cells become damaged from the exposure.

The dead skin cells dry up and start to flake and shed from the body. This cracking and flaking again deems the person an open door to infection, pain and suffering.

Chapter 4   Holistic Care for the skin

Obviously the best treatment for any disease or issue is prevention. How do you prevent skin problems?

Believe it or not one of the most simple ways is hydration. Not only of the skin but the body itself. Proper quality water intake is key to overall well being. One should consume half their body weight in water each day.

Formula example: if you weigh 150 pounds then you divide that by 2. So

150/2   = 75 . So you would drink 75 ounces of water a day.

Another easy precaution is to apply a quality, organic, petroleum from lotion or emollient. I like to use organic unrefined coconut oil. Coconut oil also possesses antibacterial properties that potentially lend more defense against pathogens.

You can add essential oils to coconut oil that   is known as carrier oil. Using a carrier oil for your essential oils topical application helps it to be used on larger areas, making it spread easier and to go further. Using a carrier oil DOES NOT dilute the effectiveness of the essential oils. A carrier oil can also be added to your vegetable capsule with your oils to tame some of the spiciness in your belly.

In the case of skin issues I would recommend the   topical application process, directly to the affected area.

Also another way to cover more of the skin's surface would be by using essential oil bath bombs in your bath water. Do your due diligence ! Not all oils are created equal! Watch for added chemicals and pollutants. The best approach is to make your own bath bombs.

Chapter 5

What Oils are beneficial for healthy skin.

Elemi, clove, Frankincense, galbanum, jasmine, and Patchouli are effective in supporting healthy skin.

For support of eczema and psoriasis support , the oils are cistus, blue cypress, Roman and German chamomile,and myrrh.

add 1 to 2 drops of desired oil diluted 50:50 to your carrier oil and apply to the affected area.

Chapter 6

Hidden dangers to the skin

One of the most insidious dangers known to not only our skin health but our overall well being something we used every day

many times a day. The chemical is known as sodium lauryl sulfate. It is put in our soaps, shampoos, body washes, dish detergents,

laundry detergents, even our toothpaste. It is what gives these products their sudsing ability, in other words their bubbling action. Sodium lauryl sulfate is a known carcinogen. Yes, the FDA knowingly allows this in our hygiene products. Please do not think for a minute it is not added to our baby products , many of them have sodium lauryl sulfate.

Do you ask yourself why there is cancer rearing its ugly head all over the place, and even in our kids? This is

one powerful reason. The skin is the largest organ of the body, so applying this harmful chemical to it affects the entire body.

The other HUGE reason is our food supply. The pesticides and chemical fertilizers being added to our food are a major source of toxicity and yes you guessed it, carcinogens. Monsanto , the manufacturer of the weed killer roundup is fully aware of the product causing lymphoma, killing off our honey bees and a boat load of other issues, yet our FDA allows it to continue. When did short term profit become more important than human life and well being?

Take heart , there are a few different ways you can help combat the toxicity being hurled at you .

The best things you can do for you and your family is

#1. maintain a clean eating meal plan.

What is clean eating?

Clean eating simply put is to eliminate processed foods from your diet all together. If it has a mother and a father or comes from the ground   eat it.

Eat Organic meat, fruits and veggies as much as you possibly can.   Grass fed pasture raised dairy provides much more of the omega 3   essential fatty acids than found in conventionally raised livestock.

In fact, eat all organic food   products as often as   possible.

Happily they offer organic coffee and tea too.

Eliminate White sugar , processed , pre-made foods, fast foods,and most breads

Sprouted bread with no added sugar is best , something like Ezekiel type brand for references purposes. There are some really good ones out there just be sure to read, read, read labels.   Watch out for added sugar in the form of corn syrup and alike.

Real organic maple syrup, local raw honey and stevia or organic agave are recommended for sweetening *

Local sourced raw honey is said to reduce allergies IE hay-fever.

*Specifically for your skin and ultimately your overall well being, use organic, sodium lauryl sulfate free products . There are some good products out there, or you can make your own with your oils, for you and your pets.

They come in dish soap, laundry detergents, body soap and shampoos and toothpastes. These can be used on your pets as well.

  Everyday pet products are containing even more and more harsh chemicals than human products.

Could this be why there is a rise in animal cancers as well?

Use your oils to make   homemade skin care products , the oils each have detoxing properties to varying degrees.

Detoxing your body at the very least weekly will help to rid the body of some of the toxins you are exposed to on a daily basis, in our air, food and such pretty much everything we encounter in today's environment.

Here is my recipe for   a detoxification bath.

Detoxing Bath:

Fill Bathtub to your preferred depth of hot water

add 15 drops of Lavender essential oil

1/4 cup of baking soda

3/4 cup of Epsom salts(also a great source of magnesium)

1/2 cup organic raw apple cider vinegar.

Mix it all in well and enjoy.

Believe me, your body will appreciate the toxins being pulled from it, while at the same time

you will feel wonderfully relaxed and refreshed.

Chapter 7

The Circulatory System and its main organs

The Heart aka the myocardium main function is to pump blood through the body to transport oxygen and nutrients to the cells. Ultimately sustaining life.

The other primary function of the heart and circulatory system is to remove wastes and carbon dioxide from the body.

The arteries are Large vessels that carry oxygenated   blood away from the heart and to the rest of the body.

Veins: Carry Deoxygenated blood from the body   back to the heart and lungs for re-oxygenation

Capillaries are the smallest of the vessels that transport blood and nutrients from the bloodstream to the cells and accept carbon dioxide and wastes from the tissues back into the bloodstream for removal from the body.

Some common issues of the circulatory system

  Heart arrhythmia. Heart arrhythmias are characterized by an abnormal beating of the heart. Sometimes a flutter can be felt in your chest(sometimes called palpitations) , such as maybe too fast a beat (>100BPM),   known as tachycardia, or perhaps too slow a beat(<60BPM) known as bradycardia.

Hardening of the arteries, or aka arteriosclerosis is when fatty plaque like substance builds up and adheres to the arterial walls and hardens. One of the main causes of hardening of the arteries is high levels of bad cholesterol known as LDL (low density lipoproteins) This can harm the body in two ways.

1.   It decreases the inside circumference of the artery,and a narrowing occurs. This may cause a decrease of the blood flow. Which in turn may result in ....the following.

2. The plaque in the arteries may break away from the arterial wall during strenuous activities resulting in a blockage of the artery (blocking the blood flow either partially or completely) which may further result in a heart attack or stroke.

Congestive heart failure is when the heart itself stops being an effective pump. The failing of the heart can be caused by damage such as occurs   from a heart attack, chronic obesity, the heart just gets tired out. The congestion is referring to excess fluid that

pools in the feet , legs, and extremities, and in chronic stages even fluid in the lungs known as pulmonary edema. This is caused by the heart's inability to adequately pump the fluids back up to the kidneys for filtering and releasing from the body.

This excess fluid puts even more strain on the heart creating a vicious cycle.

Myocardial Infarction (MI or heart attack) as mentioned before can be caused by a piece of arterial plaque detaching from the arterial wall and causing a blockage,or other times a heart attack can be caused by lack of oxygen to the myocardium which is the main muscle of the heart which causes damage to the cells from oxygen deprivation.

Chapter 8

Holistic care for the heart and circulatory system.

First and foremost as mentioned before maintain a clean eating plan.

Walking, hiking,yoga,   things like dancing if you choose and consistent exercise.

Getting adequate   intake of good fats, such as organic unrefined coconut oil, organic extra virgin olive oil , organic avocados wild caught salmon , grass fed butter etc. .

Eliminating fats that are not healthy. Trans fats, and saturated fats.   Such as those found in many processed junk foods.

A healthy intake of whole organic grains(unless you have allergies to them) and fiber as a healthy part of keeping your cholesterol in check.

Essential Oils that support the circulatory system

Goldenrod,Thyme,Marjoram,Rosemary,Peppermint,

Ylang ylang and Lavender

For support of congestive heart failure , the citrus oils such as grapefruit oil, lemon oil, tangerine oil, help support diuresing ,or in other words ridding excess fluid from the body.

Hardening of the Arteries , cassias , lavender, cypress and helichrysum are supportive oils. Cassia is thought to help regulate blood sugars which in turn will support better artery and circulatory health. Cypress strengthens the capillary walls.

Arrhythmias: lavender supports regular heart rhythms.

Recap: Circulatory System support. Clean eating diet rich in whole grains, healthy fats and consistent routine exercise and consistent

use of essential oils that support the circulatory system .

Chapter 9

The Respiratory System main organs

The lungs. The main function is the exchange of oxygen and carbon dioxide.

The lungs are made up   primarily of the bronchi, bronchioles, and Alveoli.

The bronchus is the large air transporting vessel   carrying the air from the Trachea(windpipe) into the lungs. This is what is affected when you have upper respiratory infection known as bronchitis.

The Bronchioles are smaller air carrying vessels to the alveolar sacs.

The alveolar sacs are the balloon(look like clumps of grapes) like structures that carry out the exchange of oxygen and carbon-dioxide to and from the bloodstream.

Mouth: besides nutritional intake the mouth acts as an entrance to the body for air to enter.

Nose: The job of the nose outside of a sensory organ for smelling, the noses job is to warm and filter the air that we breathe in .

Trachea is a large cartilaginous tube that takes air from the nose and mouth through Larynx (voice box) to the lungs.

The Diaphragm is a dome shaped muscle that sits between the chest cavity , also known as the thoracic cavity, and the abdominal cavity; Its function is to expand and contract the lungs like baffles, pulling air   into the lungs and pushing   the air out in a rhythmic   fashion.

A typical adult respires 18 to 20 times a minute.

The diaphragm when It's irritated and spasms   is a hiccup.

Common issues of Respiratory system.

COPD   (chronic obstructive pulmonary disease). COPD is a Long term condition that affects breathing,   it is when the air passages become obstructed   from things like   smoking , exposure to pollutants such as asbestos,heavy dust, chemicals, and Sarcoidosis, which is an inflammatory condition where the irritated cells start gathering in different areas of the lungs.   These pulmonary(lung) issues   make breathing very difficult as the lungs struggle to supply enough oxygen to the body with limited capacity.   Emphysema falls in this category.

Asthma is a condition by which the air passages of the lungs go into sudden spasm, air passages narrow and swell, making it difficult to breath in and out.

Asthma also causes excess production of mucus.

Lung cancer is when   abnormal cell growth occurs, creating tumors in or around the lungs.

The #1 cause of lung cancer is smoking tobacco products.   Both firsthand and secondhand smoke exposure.

Upper Respiratory infections or U.R.I.'s can be caused by virus,fungus or bacteria, and can range from a cold to pneumonia,influenza(flu) or even covid-19(coronavirus).

In more severe instances, things such as Tuberculosis, or sarcoidosis,tuberculosis, to name a few,   can leave lungs scarred and losing varying degrees of functionality depending on how long it goes left untreated and the damage that is sustained.

Chapter 10

Holistic Care for the respiratory system

Some of the more obvious preventative measures would be, Do Not smoke tobacco products,nor subject yourself to second hand smoke.

If you do smoke cigarettes, engage in a smoking cessation program.

Wear a mask when using solvents, pollutants, such as paints, saw dust, working on automobile brakes that contain asbestos, fiberglass, etc.

If you are prone to allergies, Peppermint and lavender are good supportive oils to use.

Eucalyptus oil helps to loosen and help raise phlegm

* FOR All Systems The   best practice is to maintain a clean eating plan*

Air purification both with oils and mechanical means as necessary.

Aerobic exercise to support lung capacity.

Meditation not only relaxes the mind and body but it also focuses on breathing and it too helps to support and expand lung capacity

 Singing and laughter also help to support lung capacity,

For lung cancer support, frankincense, lavender , alkaline diet and removing ALL sugar from diet. It is believed that cancer can not survive in an alkaline body and it needs sugar to thrive

Detox bath as mentioned in the chapters before.

Use homemade cleaning products that are chemical free such as those made with essential oils to prevent irritation to your lungs as well as your pets lungs. Remember they are much closer to the floor than we are.

For URI support,   Oregano, thyme and eucalyptus oils are supportive of these issues. Also citrus fruits with vitamin C to boost the immune system.

Oils that support the Respiratory system are thyme eucalyptus,frankincense,palo santo,sandalwood, Clove and Hyssop

Chapter 11

Nervous and musculoskeletal system major organs.

The bones form the skeletal system whose main function is to maintain the form of the body and to enable movement, stature and to protect the internal organs of the body from injury.

Cartilage Acts as a "shock absorber" between adults bones, it also allows free movements in the joints.

Muscles: There are two types of muscles striated and smooth muscle, their main function is movement.

Both cardiac and smooth muscle   are involuntary , in other words they function without thought required. Example the beating of your heart.

Skeletal   muscle is voluntary, whereas it requires conscious thought to move it.

Tendons main function is to attach the skeletal muscles of the body   to the bones of the skeleton.

Ligaments main function is to connect bone to bone.

Nerves connect the brain, spinal cord and sensory organs to the rest of the body. Providing sight, hearing, touch, taste, ability to smell and physical movement.

Brain is the central processor for the entirety of the body. Thought, vision, sound, tactile(touch) , and smells are all interpreted within the brain.

Memory, learning, all happen in the cerebrum.

The Cerebellum, the   smaller portion of the brain is located at the back of the skull controls balance and movement.

The Brainstem Consists of the midbrain, the ponds ,and the medulla oblongata. It controls the involuntary or parasympathetic   nervous system functions ; such as breathing, heart beat, fight or flight reactions. IE. things that do not require thought to occur.

Spinal cord ,The brain and the spinal cord make up the part of the body known and the central nervous system.

The spinal cord carries electrical impulses from the brain to the body and visa versa creating movement, sensations etc.

Sensory organs Eyes, Ears,Nose, Tongue-taste,Tactile- touch and the 6th sense is intuition

Chapter 12

Common Musculoskeletal- nervous system

Possible issues:

Paralysis: Loss of use due trauma and severance of spinal cord or degenerative neurological disease.

Neuropathy: Inflammatory nerve condition, most common diabetic causing burning, stabbing pain, numbness, tingling in any one or all of the following, the hands, feet and legs. Makes one more susceptible to injury due to decreased sensation in feet and legs.

Wintergreen and frankincense help support relief of symptoms.

Tendinitis : inflammation of the tendon , painful and can temporarily limit the range of motion in the area affected.

Wintergreen,Frankenstein and Copaiba help support tendinitis ease.

Alzheimer's: severe loss of memory, thought to stem from amyloid deposits on the brain and possibly fluorides effect on the pineal gland.

Frankincense, clary sage , Hawaiian sandalwood help to detox the pineal gland. Also use the detox bath protocol as well.

Other Oils that Support

Cedarwood,German chamomile,Roman Chamomile,Frankincense,Ginger,Lavender and clary sage.

Chapter 13

The digestive system and basic endocrine systems major organs.

Mouth-Salivary glands

The mouth,other than to speak and breathe ,is the first step in digesting. The teeth provide a grinding motion which grinds food up for easier digestion.

Salivary Glands produce moisture for food for ease of swallowing but also contain digestive enzymes that go to work on digesting carbohydrates immediately. The

Tongue moves the food about in the mouth for more even chewing, it also pushes the food to the back of the mouth for swallowing.

The esophagus,sometimes called the food tube, is the vehicle that makes a squeezing motion called peristalsis   that basically transports the food from the throat down to the stomach.

The stomach, A larger J shaped organ that accepts the food from the esophagus . The stomach pummels the food down further into liquid form called chyme.   The stomach receives digestive enzymes from the liver and pancreas and the stomach produces hydrochloric acid that helps with breaking down food.

The liver is located under the right rib cage. It produces bile that is stored in the gallbladder for the digestion of fats,   but the liver also has the Important role of producing prothrombin and fibrinogen , the two main factors responsible for causing blood to clot.   The liver is

a major component in metabolizing many of the pharmaceuticals and alcohol consumed.

The pancreas , The pancreas produces pancreatic enzymes that aid in   digestion but is mostly known for its   role in insulin production . Insulin is a substance that pushes the glucose and nutrition, across the cell membrane.   When there is not enough insulin , the cells do not get properly nourished, and the glucose floats around in the bloodstream unused. High and low blood sugar levels alike are dangerous for your body, primarily from malnourished cells from the lack of insulin. High blood sugars , or hyperglycemia , is one of the major causes of plaque build up and hardening of the arteries according to modern day experts

The intestines are composed of the duodenum, the jejunum and ileum,are considered the *small intestine.* The cecum, ascending colon , transverse, descending, sigmoid, rectum and anus are the parts known as the *large colon* .

The small intestines add a large part in absorbing the digested nutrients for the body's use .

The large intestines carry waste products to evacuate from the body, but also play a role in the control of water levels in the body by retaining or releasing water into the bowel tract.

Chapter 14

Most common issues of the digestive and endocrine system.

Ulcers both in the stomach and intestines.

An ulcer is an open raw area in the stomach, esophagus or intestinal wall. Some ulcers are   caused by a poor diet, bacterial causation such as H-Pylori , alcohol consumption, cigarette smoking and stress to name a few. To support a healthy GI tract, maintain a healthy clean organic diet. You may add organic raw apple cider vinegar to help with acid content(check with health care provider first).Be sure to consume an adequate amount of roughage in your diet, fiber, such as organic whole grains, greens, and other fruits and vegetables , especially raw as they are living food and still contain alkalizing enzymes. Also utilize the oils to be listed below.

Acid Reflux   Use the same protocol as above but also you may wish to abstain from   eating for at least one hour before going to bed to prevent worsening symptoms of GERD(gastroesophageal reflux disease).

For constipation issues,   ensure you have adequate fluid intake as mentioned in the aforementioned chapters.

  Again maintain a diet full or organic healthy fruits and vegetables

Diarrhea and Irritable bowel all respond in similar ways to the the same protocol

Hepatitis is a condition where as the liver becomes diseased and inflamed, It can be chronic and it can be fatal .

There are different kinds of hepatitis. More common ones are ,A, B, and C.

Hepatitis A is viral,

Hep.B can be spread by bodily fluids, as with in sexual intercourse,blood and saliva with an infected person.

  Hep.C   is exclusively   blood to blood contact with an infected person.

Diabetes type I and type II

Type 1 is a prediabetic state whereas the blood test known as a hemoglobin A1C determines what the blood sugar levels over the past 3 months have averaged. A test score of > 6.5 deems you a diabetic.

This condition is usually caused by sedentary lifestyles, lack of consistent exercise, poor diet, consisting primarily of processed foods and refined sugars.

There is no blame here, The USA is considered one of the most unhealthy diets in the world, containing the highest amounts of added sugar, and refined processed ingredients. Take a look at the ingredients on your grocery items, I encourage you , that if you can not pronounce most of the list of ingredients DON'T EAT IT!

Type 1 diabetes   is sometimes known as insulin resistance. This often may be a precursor to type II diabetes . Type 1 can often be reversed with consistent healthy diet and exercise.

Type II diabetes usually requires medical intervention of some sort. In most cases western medicine   Dr's prescribe drugs like sulfonaureas that stimulate the pancreas to produce more insulin which in turn should help better control insulin levels. Diabetes type II can lead to many related illnesses , blindness, kidney failure, heart attack and strokes therefore diabetes should be taken very seriously.

Cassia and cinnamon are essential   oils known to support healthier blood sugar levels.

Again   healthy organic whole grains, vegetables and lean organic meats would be a good diet plan to follow. Fruits at this point may need to be limited to berries, such as blue, black , red and black raspberries, as well as fresh strawberries which are lower in sugar and carbs at around 6 Grams of carbs per half cup serving.

Diabetes Specific support oils

Clove

Coriander

Fennel

Dill

Octea

Cinnamon

Lemongrass

Obviously remove all refined white sugar and products with sugar in them. Use organic Stevia for sweetening as often as possible.

Adhere to the clean eating plan . Do not eat white pasta, bread and such. if you wish to on the occasion imbibe in some bread a good recommendation again is a sprouted whole grain bread. Do your due diligence and check the labels for hidden sugars and avoid them. Low carbohydrate is a good plan to follow especially when trying to regain control of your blood sugars and lose the extra pounds you need to shed as a rule of thumb keeping your carbohydrate intake 30 Grams a day or less and Exercise at least three times a week. Walking, hiking, biking , dancing whatever you fancy.

   ***Please check with your primary care practitioner before beginning any changes in eating plans or any exercise plan. ***

Key Points

Maintain a healthy clean eating diet

May add Raw apple cider vinegar to alkalize your body 30cc a day

Eat a diet rich in organic grains , fruits and veggies to add adequate supply of fiber to help maintain bowel regularity, unless doing low carb, omit grains and most fruits, all breads, and all sugars.

Make sure to maintain hydration , water intake helps keep bowels regular .

Maintain a regular exercise routine .A sedentary lifestyle can cause issues with constipation.

Chapter 15 Genital-Urinary system major organs

Kidneys,the main function of the kidney is to filter out impurities from the blood , help maintain the body's sodium levels, fluid levels, blood pressure and beyond.

The urinary bladder is an elastic like , flexible organ that holds the urine until it is ready to be released from the body.

Ureters are a pair of tube-like structures that drain the urine from the kidney and take it to the urinary bladder.

The urethra is a smaller tube structure that takes urine from the bladder out of the body, though it is a longer structure in the male body, the entire length of penis.

The Urinary meatus is the spherical muscle that expands and contracts to release the urine from the body by controlling the opening and closing of the opening .

The Penis is the male sexual organ that houses the urethra, and transports both urine and seaman from the urinary bladder and the seminal vesicles respectfully, to the outside of the body

The Vagina is the canal that connects the uterus to the outside of the body. It is also known as the birth canal.

It is the receptacle for seamen in the reproductive process.

The Fallopian tubes are the tubial structures that carry the egg from the ovaries to the uterus.

The Ovaries a pair of round nickel sized organs sitting to the left and right top of the uterus   that hold a woman's   ovum or   eggs they release one egg once a month during a woman's menstrual years

The Uterus is the pear sized organ that incubates the human fetus

The Adrenal glands are stocking cap shaped glands that sit on top of the kidneys. The   major function is to produce hormones that help regulate your blood pressure, immune system, metabolism, response to stress such as secreting adrenaline, and cortisol as well as other needed functions.

The Scrotum is the sac of skin that houses and protects the testicles.

Testicles are Also known as the male gonads. Their major role is 1,to produce sperm for reproduction and they also secrete hormones , such as testosterone that give men their male characteristics such as beard, lower voices,   and as a rule more muscular than women.

Chapter 16 the

Most common issues of the   G.U. system.

For the Ovary , Fallopian tubes,and vagina

Genital yeast infection is characterized by burning , itching and often a cottage cheese like vaginal discharge is present.

Suggestions,   Pre and probiotics, eating organic live cultured sugar free Greek yogurt and detox baths.

Lavender, peppermint and lemongrass have antifungal properties (yeast is a fungus). I would suggest putting them in a carrier oil and then in your bath as these oils on mucus membranes can be pretty spicy and burn(sting).

Sexually transmitted diseases.

Suggestions,   obviously protected sex with the use of a condom will   in most cases help prevent the transmission of pathogens though it is not full proof.

Endometriosis is an overgrowth of endometrial tissues, causing pain, heavy cramping, hard menstrual flow. The endometrial tissue , in the worst case scenario can actually attach to the bowels, bladder and pelvic wall.

Cervical, uterine or ovarian cancer:

  Any and all cancers can be resisted to varying degrees, with an organic clean eating plan, alkaline foods, detoxing by way of baths, there are cleansing protocols for diet detoxification. Limit all sugar intake and as with your clean eating, removing all processed foods and refined sugars will support a healthy body.

Also routine pap smears are a good way for early detection of issues.

Tubal pregnancies are when the fertilized egg from the female does not make it to the uterus to attach to the uterine wall, instead it adheres to the Fallopian tube . When this occurs it is life threatening, the possibility of the tube rupturing as the embryo starts to grow creates hemorrhaging. With potentially extensive blood loss and at times leading to death.

Polycystic ovary disease is characterized by fluid filled cysts growing on the ovaries.

This can be quite painful and can be considered a cause of metabolic syndrome and insulin resistance. A low carb diet has been suggested will straighten out the metabolic resistance,also regaining blood sugar control.

Kidney and bladder

Kidney and bladder infection is a bacterial or fungal entrance to the otherwise sterile urinary tract. It is usually characterized by burning, painful difficult urination and at times there will be the presence of hematuria will be present(blood in the urine). Staying hydrated is a crucial component , aiding the bladder and urethra in flushing out possible pathogens. Urinating before and after sexual intercourse helps support flushing of bacteria exchanged during sex.

Kidney stones are calcifications that grow in the kidneys, they can range from sandy grit to grape sized stones. They are extremely painful and probably the closest a man will ever come to knowing what childbirth feels like. At times the larger stones will need to be surgically removed so not to cause kidney damage as the stone blocks the ureter and does not allow the urine to drain from the kidney.

Citrus oils   IE grapefruit essential oil helps support the rounding off of the rough edges of the stones, potentially allowing them to pass more freely.

Neurogenic bladder   is when the nerves to the bladder become damaged. The damage may stem from spinal cord injuries, diabetes and other neurological disorders. When you have a neurogenic bladder, you may experience incontinence, difficulty starting a stream and many shades of gray in between.   The preventative kind which stems from Uncontrolled diabetes , could potentially be avoided by maintaining good blood sugar control . A healthy blood sugar level range is 80-120 mg/dl.

My go to oil for anything neurological is Frankincense essential oil.

Chapter 17

Oils that Support the g-u system

Female specific:
Melissa,Sage,Vetiver,Yarrow and Ylang ylang

(Male) hormone imbalance: Rosemary, sage, fennel, geranium frankincense,Clary sage

Key Points

Routine pap smears.

Routine prostate exams.

Protected sex to prevent sexually transmitted diseases.

Organic soaps, body washes, that are sodium lauryl sulfate free. As well as aluminum free deodorants.

Organic Clean eating plan.

Avoid talcum powders, including baby powder. Check carefully for talc as an ingredient it is a known carcinogen   also has been found to have traces of asbestos which is another known carcinogen

About the author

Hi, I am Janie Howe. It is a pleasure to have you as a student. It is my passion to love and teach others who are seeking information to live a better, happier, healthy life .

I have a strong medical background with a 30 year nursing career under my belt. I retired about 15 years ago from nursing when at that time I became very interested in Holistic medicine and alternative treatment modalities.   I was introduced by a dear friend to Reiki in 2009 as well as Essential oils. I soon became Reiki certified and 3 years after my first certification I became a certified Reiki Master teacher, an essential oils specialist   and have had the privilege of serving in this capacity for over   a decade and loving every minute of it.

I also studied and became an Tony Robbins strategic interventionist, results driven coach, an advanced Ho'Oponopono practitioner certified by Dr. Joe Vitale, as well as   A Law of Attraction facilitator. I studied the Psychology of eating , and am currently a student of life with Robert Tennyson Stevens.

I love to teach and share the things that I have learned and found to help me live a more joyous and abundant life. I wrote a book dedicated to the sharing of much of this knowledge Entitled " The Portal in the Park, the teachings of Brown Feather" By Janie Rose, which if you want to learn in   more about the Law of Attraction, told in an entertaining way, you will find it on Amazon.com , and Balboa Publishing . Com.

I look forward to many years of sharing and caring and growing with you,my beloved students, friends and family . Blessings of Love and light to all who seek it. I vote for your Victory . I am your permanent Victory in the light.

                                        Always,
        Jane

                If you wish to explore my oils of Choice ,
you may learn more at www.youngliving.com   Please
if you would like to become a part of the Young living
essential oils family, My member number is 1074037 .